Your Menopause Wellness Guide: Welcome to **"THE 7-DAY MENOPAUSE DIET,"** your go-to resource for navigating menopause with confidence and vitality. I'm here to share practical tips, easy recipes, and helpful insights to support your journey to better health. **Why this book?** It's all about sharing what works, making life more straightforward, and helping you feel your best during menopause. Think of me as your no-nonsense ally, here to offer concrete advice and tasty solutions for a happier menopausal experience. As we dive into these pages, picture a plate filled with colorful veggies, lean proteins, and wholesome grains - all designed to boost your hormonal health and energy levels. Each chapter is a roadmap to feeling good and eating well, from intelligent food choices to mindful eating habits. Prepare for a week-long adventure of nourishing meals, practical tips, and a sprinkle of self-care. So, roll up your sleeves, grab a grocery list, and let's get cooking! Together, we'll explore delicious recipes, easy strategies, and simple steps to make your menopausal journey healthier and happier. It's time to dive in, enjoy the process, and embrace a menopause filled with delicious discoveries. Let's make wellness a way of life. Let's get started! In this menopause wellness guide, you'll find practical advice and delicious recipes to support you through this transformative phase of life. From easy meal ideas to handy tips, this book is your companion for embracing well-being during menopause. Get ready to discover the power of nutrient-rich foods like vibrant fruits, hearty vegetables, and lean proteins that can fuel your body and nourish your hormones. These ingredients are not just for taste; they are your allies in promoting hormonal balance and sustained energy throughout your menopausal journey. As we journey through each chapter, you'll learn how to make simple yet impactful changes in your eating habits, encouraging mindful choices that nourish your body and mind. Say goodbye to overwhelm and hello to practical solutions that fit seamlessly into your daily routine, making wellness an achievable and enjoyable goal. So, grab a pen to jot down your favorites, dust off your apron, and dive into a week of rejuvenating meals that will energize and inspire you. This is your road map to a healthier, happier menopause - one plate at a time. Let's embark on this culinary adventure together and create a new chapter of well-being and vitality in your menopausal story.

Cutting Out The Bad Foods

Cutting out processed foods, refined carbohydrates, dairy products, and other hormone-disrupting foods from recipes can help reset hormonal balance and promote overall well-being.

Processed foods: To promote hormonal balance, avoid processed foods such as packaged snacks, sugary breakfast cereals, processed meats, fast food, frozen meals, and sugary drinks. Opt for whole, nutrient-dense foods like fruits, vegetables, lean proteins, and healthy fats.

Refined carbohydrates: In menopause, it is advisable to avoid refined carbohydrates such as white bread, white rice, sugary cereals, and pastries, as they can spike blood sugar levels and disrupt hormone balance. Opt for whole grains like quinoa, brown rice, oats, and whole wheat bread for more stable energy levels and better hormonal health.

Highly processed vegetable oils: In menopause, it is recommended to avoid highly processed vegetable oils such as soybean oil, corn oil, sunflower oil, and canola oil, as they can contribute to inflammation and hormonal imbalances. Instead, choose healthier alternatives like olive, coconut, and avocado oil for better hormonal health and overall well-being.

Dairy products: During menopause, avoid full-fat dairy products like whole milk and cheese to help balance hormones. Choose low-fat or non-dairy options such as almond milk and tofu-based cheeses for better hormone health.

Alcohol: Avoiding alcohol during menopause is advised as it can worsen symptoms like hot flashes and sleep disturbances by disrupting hormone balance. Removing alcohol from your diet can help improve menopausal symptoms and support hormonal health. An odd cheeky one won't harm you!

Caffeine: Avoiding caffeine during menopause is beneficial as it can trigger hot flashes, worsen insomnia, and contribute to hormonal imbalances. Reducing caffeine can help relieve menopausal symptoms and promote better sleep quality and hormonal stability during this phase.

Sugary drinks: Avoiding sugary drinks during menopause is vital as they can lead to blood sugar spikes, weight gain, and hormonal imbalances. Opting for water, herbal teas, or infused waters instead of sugary beverages can help manage menopausal symptoms and support overall hormonal health during this stage of life.

Replacing these foods with whole,nutrient-dense options like fruits, vegetables, lean proteins, and healthy fats can support hormone balance. Always consult with a healthcare professional before making significant dietary changes.

In this chapter, readers will discover the power of nutrient-dense foods to support hormone balance and boost energy levels during menopause.

Incorporating fruits and vegetables rich in antioxidants and vitamins is essential to promote hormonal health.

Fruits: Berries (blueberries, strawberries, raspberries), citrus fruits (oranges, lemons), avocado, and apples.

Vegetables: Leafy greens (spinach, kale, Swiss chard), calciferous vegetables (broccoli, cauliflower, Brussels sprouts), bell peppers, and sweet potatoes.

They are all excellent choices for supporting hormonal balance and overall health during menopause.

Exploring lean proteins as a critical source of essential amino acids for hormone production and energy.

Lean Proteins: Salmon, chicken breast, turkey, tofu, lentils, and beans.

Embracing healthy fats like avocados and nuts to aid in hormone regulation and overall vitality.

Healthy Fats: Avocado, nuts (almonds, walnuts), seeds (flaxseeds, chia seeds), olive oil, and coconut oil.

Delving into the benefits of whole grains and complex carbohydrates for sustained energy levels and hormone support

Whole Grains: Quinoa, brown rice, oats, wheat bread, and barley.

Incorporating various foods into your diet can help support hormone balance and promote overall well-being during menopause.

This chapter offers structured meal plans for **breakfast, lunch,** and **dinner** to support menopausal health, weight management, and overall well-being. Readers will learn how to create nutritious and satisfying meals that cater to their dietary needs and promote a healthy lifestyle.

Following the menu plans for breakfast, lunch, and dinner with well-chosen snacks, you can effectively maintain steady energy levels throughout **the seven-day menopause diet.** Starting your day with a hormone-balancing breakfast, fueling with nutrient-rich lunch options, and winding down with satisfying dinner choices, complemented by healthy snacks, ensures a continuous energy source to support you throughout the day. As you progress through the week, you will likely notice a significant boost in your energy levels, feeling revitalized and more energized as your body receives the nourishment it needs for optimal function. This structured approach to meal planning fuels your body and helps maintain hormonal balance, leaving you feeling invigorated and empowered to take on each day with vitality and resilience.

BREAKFAST OPTIONS

Breakfast Options: Explore a variety of breakfast recipes that provide energy and nourishment to kick-start the day

Avocado Toast with Poached Egg.

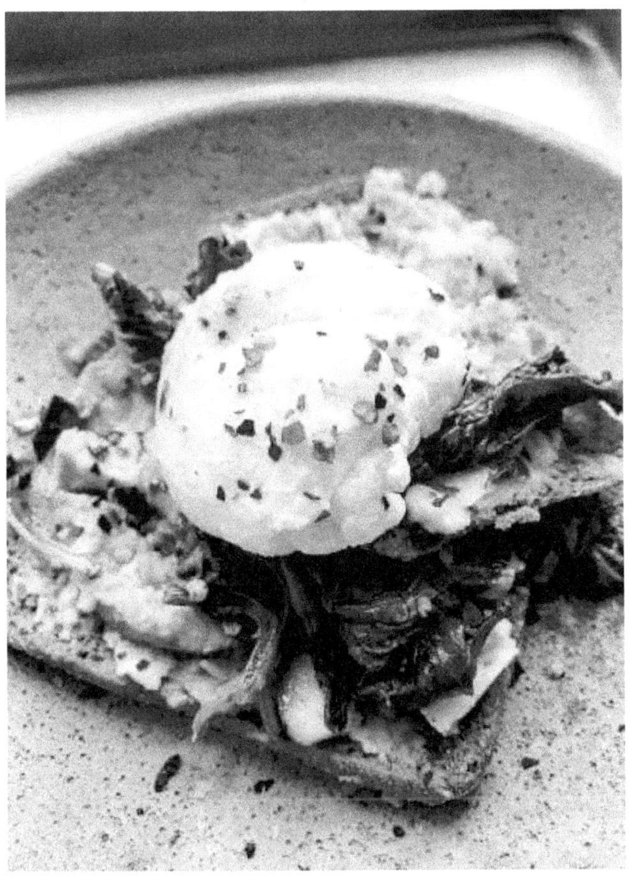

Season with salt and pepper, and add optional toppings like cherry tomatoes, spinach-crumbled feta cheese, or a sprinkle of red pepper flakes.

Greek Yogurt Parfait.

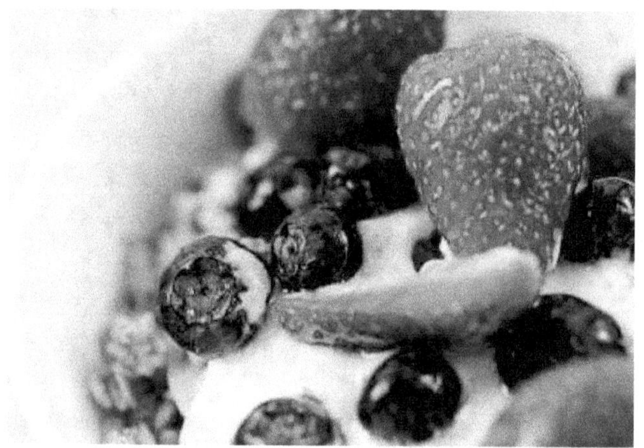

Ingredients:

1 cup Greek yogurt

1/2 cup Granola Mixed berries (blueberries, strawberries)

Drizzle Honey or maple syrup

Instructions:

Layer Greek yogurt, granola, and mixed berries in a glass bowl.

Repeat the layers until the container is filled to your liking.

Drizzle honey or maple syrup on top for added sweetness.

Enjoy this creamy and fruity parfait for a satisfying and nutritious breakfast.

Spinach and Feta Omelette

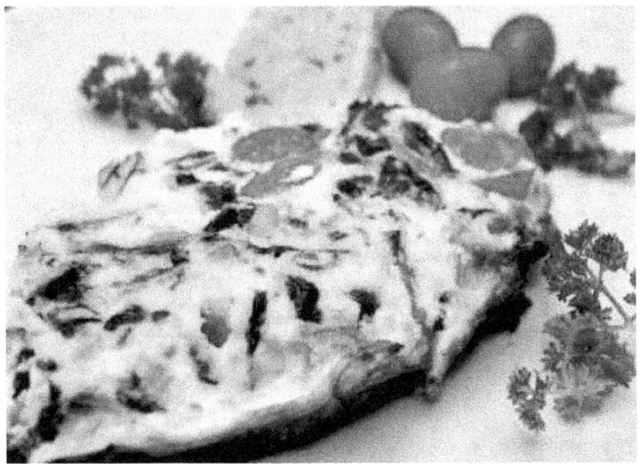

Ingredients:

2 eggs

Handful of fresh spinach

1/4 cup of Crumbled feta cheese

Salt and pepper

1 tbsp Olive oil

Instructions:

Beat the eggs in a bowl and season with salt and pepper.

Heat olive oil in a pan and sauté the spinach until wilted.

Pour the beaten eggs over the spinach and cook until the edges are set.

Sprinkle feta cheese on one half of the omelet, fold over the other half, and cook until the cheese melts.

Serve this flavorful and protein-packed omelet for a hearty breakfast option.

Berry Banana Smoothie Bowl.

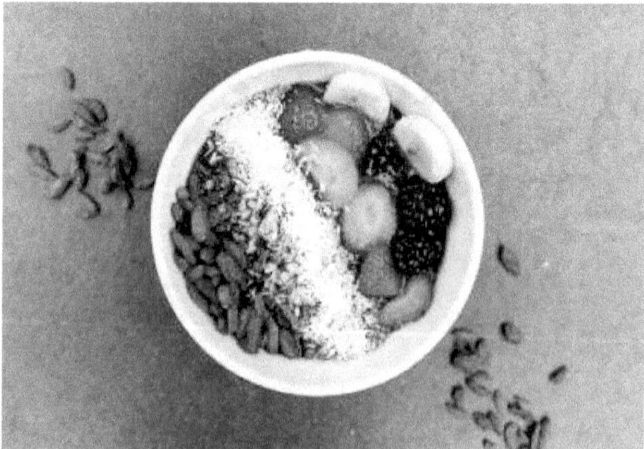

Ingredients:

1 frozen banana

1/2 cup mixed berries (such as blueberries, raspberries)

1/2 cup almond milk

Toppings:

Instructions:

Blend the frozen banana, mixed berries, and almond milk until smooth.

Pour the smoothie into a bowl.

Top with sliced banana, granola, and chia seeds.

Enjoy this refreshing and nourishing smoothie bowl.

Banana Protein Smoothie

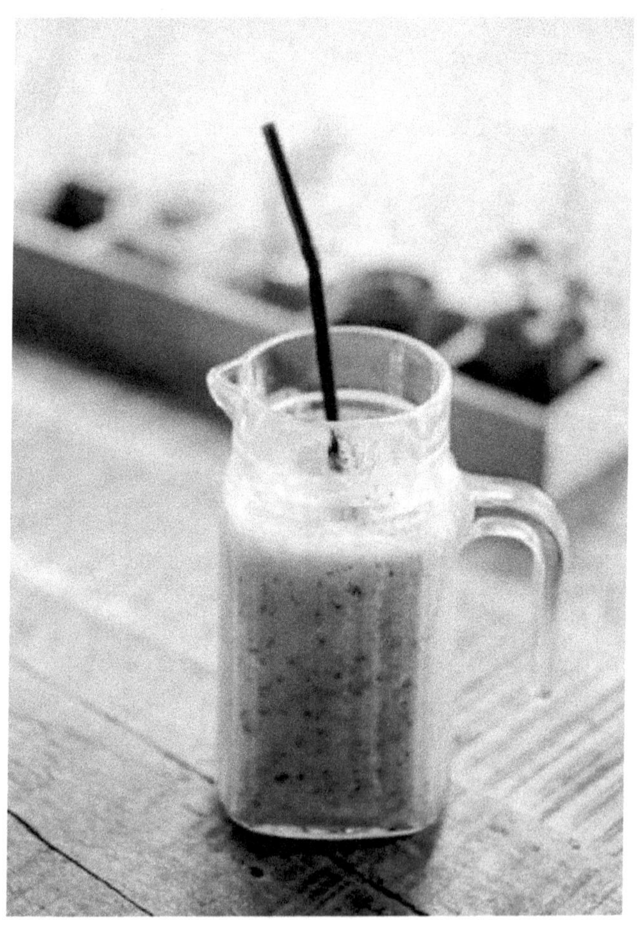

Ingredients:

1 ripe banana

1 scoop of your favorite protein powder (such as whey, plant-based, or collagen)

1 cup almond milk (or any milk of your choice)

1 tbsp almond butter (or peanut butter)

1/2 tsp cinnamon

Ice cubes (optional)

Instructions:

Prepare Ingredients:

Peel the banana and break it into chunks for more effortless blending.

Blend the Smoothie:

In a blender, combine the banana chunks, protein powder, almond milk, almond butter, and cinnamon.

Add a few ice cubes if you prefer a colder smoothie.

Blend until smooth and creamy. Add more almond milk to reach your desired consistency if the smoothie is too thick.

Overnight Chia Seed Pudding.

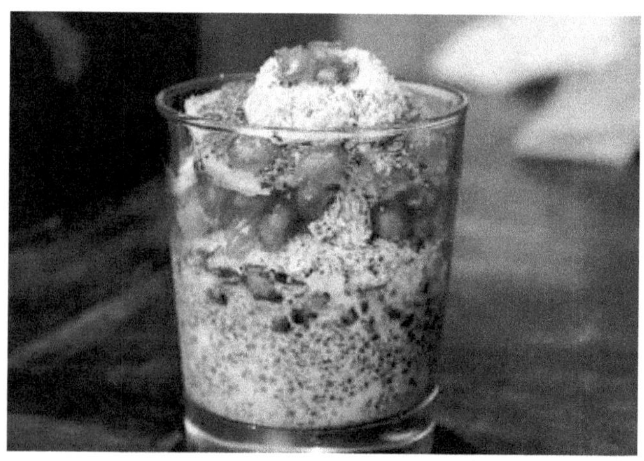

Ingredients:

2 tbsp chia seeds

1/2 cup Almond Milk

1/2 tsp vanilla extract

Sliced fruit (such as strawberries, pomegranate)

Honey or maple syrup (optional)

Instructions:

Mix chia seeds, almond milk, and vanilla extract in a bowl.

Refrigerate the mixture overnight to allow the chia seeds to thicken.

Serve the pudding in the morning, top with sliced fruit, and drizzle with honey or maple syrup if desired.

Enjoy this creamy and satisfying chia seed pudding for a nutritious breakfast.

Oatmeal with Sliced Banana and Chia Seeds.

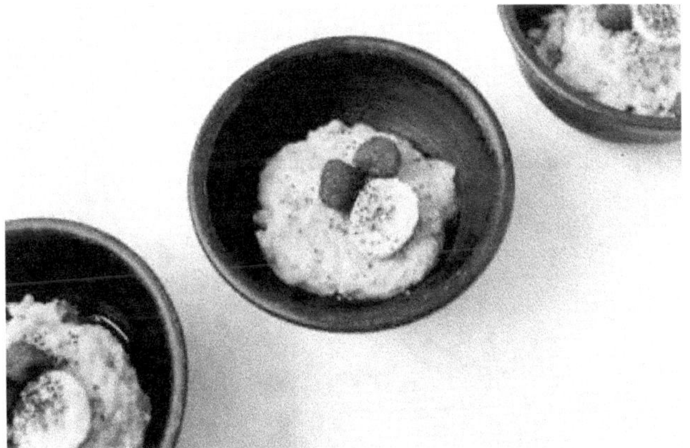

Ingredients:

1/2 cup oats

1 cup water or milk

1/2 banana, sliced

1 tbsp chia seeds

Instructions:

In a saucepan, bring water or milk to a boil.

Add oats and cook according to package instructions.

Once cooked, top with sliced banana and sprinkle with chia seeds for added nutrition and texture.

Serve warm and enjoy a hearty breakfast to start your day.

Scrambled Eggs with Sauteed Spinach and Whole Grain Toast.

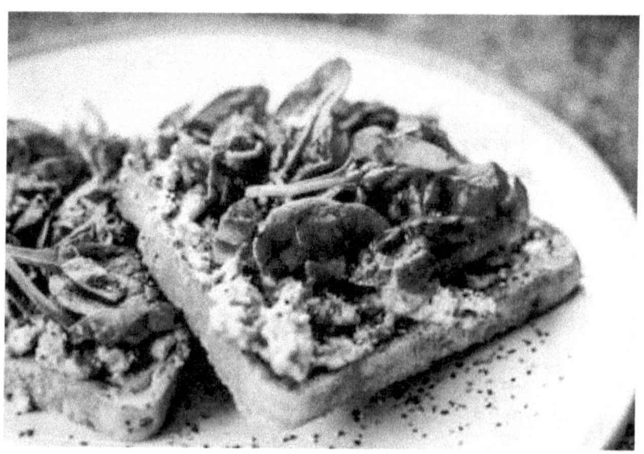

Ingredients:

2 eggs

1 cup fresh spinach

1 slice of whole-grain toast

1 tbsp Olive oil

Salt and pepper

Instructions:

Saute spinach in a pan with olive oil until wilted.

Whisk eggs in a bowl, season with salt and pepper, and scramble in the same pan as the spinach.

Serve the scrambled eggs with sauteed spinach on whole grain toast.

Green Smoothie Bowl.

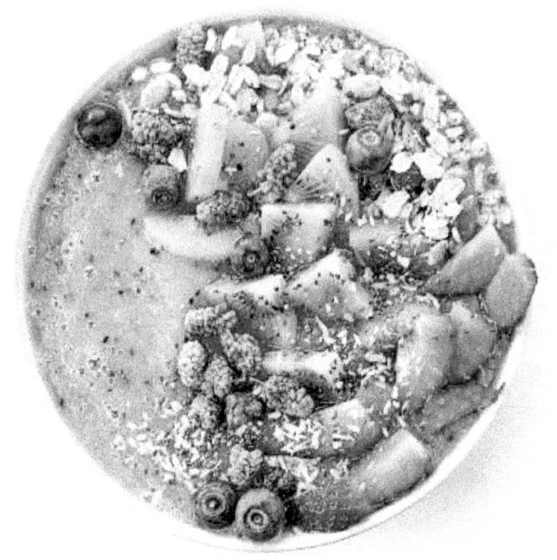

Ingredients:

1 cup spinach

1/2 cup frozen mixed berries

1/2 banana

1/2 cup almond milk

1 tbsp chia seeds

Toppings:

Granola, coconut flakes, sliced kiwi

Instructions:

Blend spinach, mixed berries, banana, and almond milk until smooth.

Pour the smoothie into a bowl and top with chia seeds, granola, coconut flakes, and sliced kiwi.

Greek yogurt with nuts and berries.

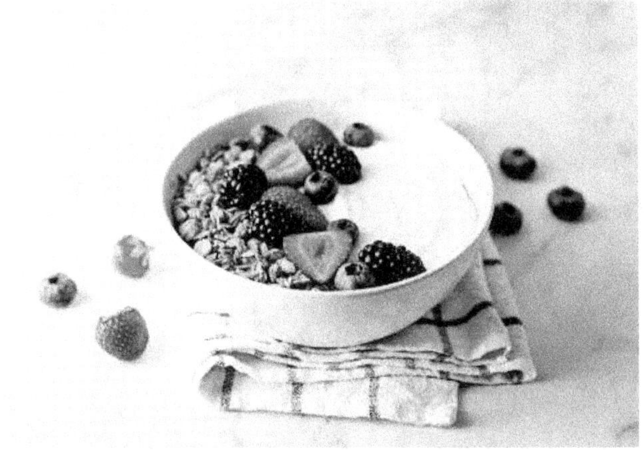

Ingredients:

1/2 cup Greek yogurt

Assorted berries (blueberries, strawberries, raspberries)Mixed nuts (almonds, walnuts)

Instructions:

In a bowl, add Greek yogurt as the base.

Top with assorted berries and mixed nuts for added flavor and texture.

Enjoy this nutritious and filling breakfast option.

Whole Grain Toast with Ricotta Cheese and Sliced Strawberries.

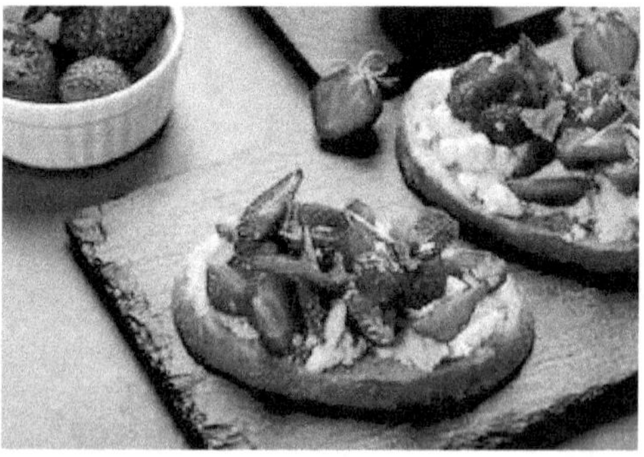

Ingredients:

1 slice of sourdough bread

2 tbsp ricotta cheese

Sliced strawberries

Drizzle of honey (optional)

Instructions:

Toast the whole grain bread until crispy.

Spread ricotta cheese on the toast.

Top with sliced strawberries and drizzle with honey for added sweetness.

These recipes offer diverse and delicious options to kick-start your day with flavor and nourishment.

LUNCH OPTIONS

Lunch Ideas: Discover delicious and balanced lunch options that support satiety and help maintain energy levels throughout the day.

Quinoa and Chickpea Salad

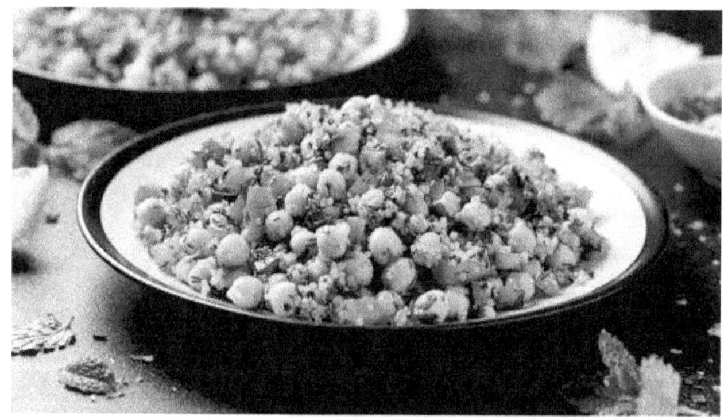

Ingredients:

1 cup cooked quinoa

1/2 cup canned chickpeas, rinsed and drained

1/4 Cherry tomatoes, halved

1/4 Cucumber, diced

1/4 Red onion, thinly sliced

Fresh parsley, chopped

Lemon vinaigrette dressing

Feta cheese (optional)

Salt and pepper to taste

Instructions

Combine a bowl of quinoa, chickpeas, cherry tomatoes, cucumber, red onion, and parsley.

Drizzle with lemon vinaigrette dressing and toss to combine.

Season with salt and pepper, and top with crumbled feta cheese if desired.

Enjoy this flavorful and protein-packed salad.

Turkey Avocado Wrap

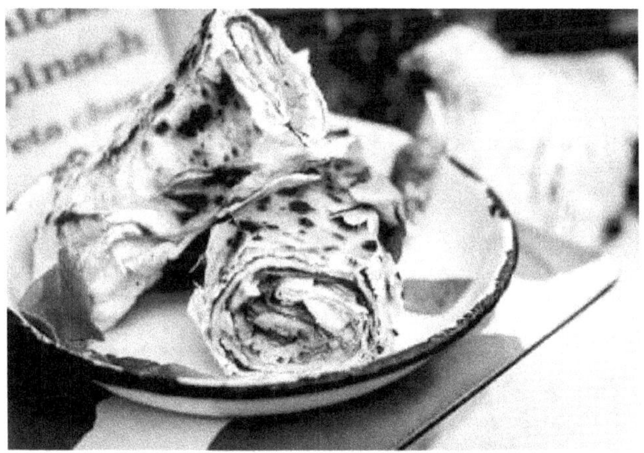

Ingredients:

Sliced turkey breast

1 Avocado, mashed

2 Whole grain wrap or tortilla

1 cup Spinach leaves

1/2 cup Roasted red peppers

Mustard or hummus

Salt and pepper to taste

Instructions:

Spread mashed avocado on the wrap.

Layer sliced turkey, spinach leaves, roasted red peppers, and a drizzle of mustard or hummus.

Season with salt and pepper, wrap it up and slice in half for a satisfying and easy-to-eat lunch.

Lentil and Vegetable Soup

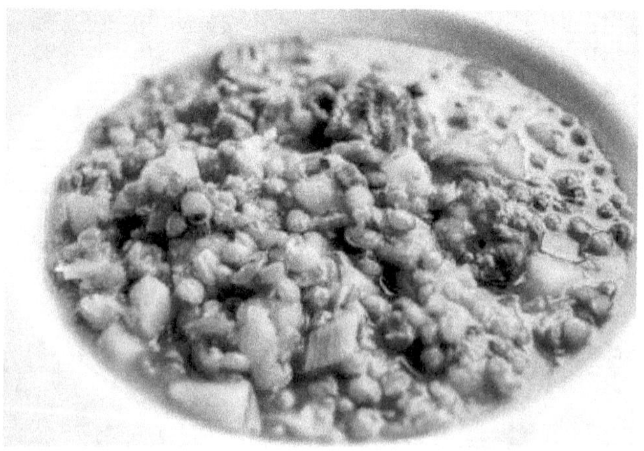

Ingredients:

1 cup cooked lentils

2 cups Mixed vegetables (carrots, celery, potatoes)

Vegetable broth

2 Garlic, minced

1 tsp Herbs (such as thyme and rosemary)

Salt and pepper to taste

Instructions:

In a pot, saute garlic and vegetables until softened.

Add lentils, vegetable broth, herbs, salt, and pepper.

Simmer until the flavors meld together and the soup is heated through.

Enjoy this hearty and comforting soup for a nourishing lunch option.

Continue to the following message for more lunch recipes.

Chicken Avocado Salad

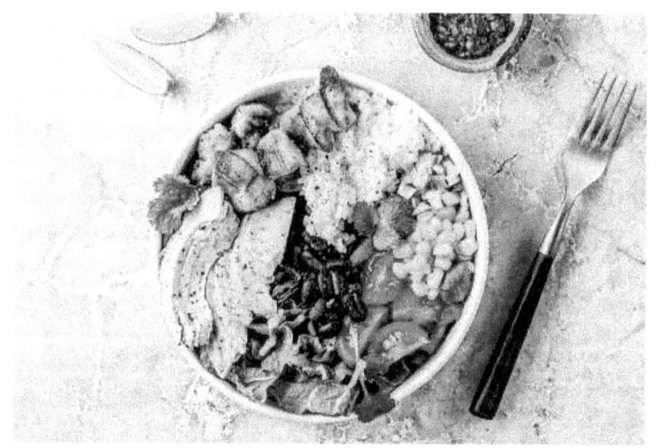

Ingredients:

Grilled chicken breast, sliced

1/2 cup Romaine lettuce, chopped

1/2 cup Cherry tomatoes, halved

1 Avocado, diced

1/2 cup Cucumber, sliced

1/4 cup Red onion, thinly sliced

1 tbsp Balsamic vinaigrette dressing

Instructions:

Combine the grilled chicken, lettuce, cherry tomatoes, avocado, cucumber, and red onion in a bowl.

Drizzle with balsamic vinaigrette dressing and toss to coat.

Serve this refreshing chicken avocado salad for a protein-packed and flavorful lunch option.

Tuna Nicoise Salad:

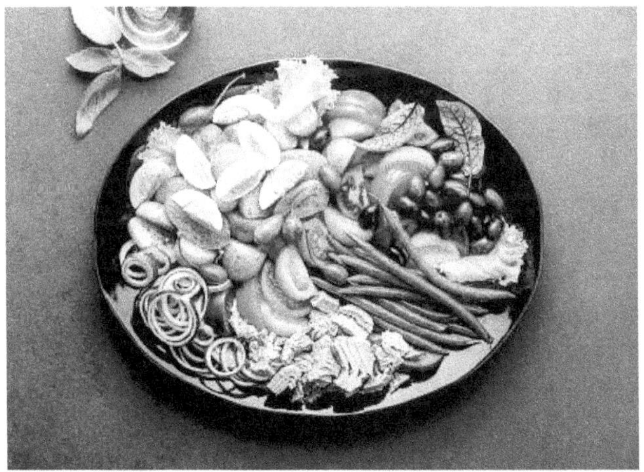

Ingredients:

1 can tuna, drained

1/2 cup small red potatoes, halved

2 eggs

1/2 cup green beans, trimmed

1 cup cherry tomatoes, halved

1/4 cup Niçoise olives

2 tbsp capers

4 cups mixed greens

salt and pepper to taste

For the vinaigrette:

1/4 cup olive oil

2 tbsp red wine vinegar

1 tsp Dijon mustard

1 clove garlic, minced

salt and pepper to taste

Instructions:

Boil Potatoes and Eggs:

In a pot of boiling water, cook the potatoes until tender, about 12-15 minutes.

In the same pot, add the eggs and cook for 8-10 minutes for hard-boiled eggs.

Once done, peel and quarter the eggs.

Prepare Green Beans:

Blanch the green beans in a separate pot of boiling water for 2-3 minutes until bright green and crisp-tender.

Transfer to an ice bath to stop cooking.

Make the Vinaigrette:

To make the vinaigrette, whisk together olive oil, red wine vinegar, Dijon mustard, garlic, salt, and pepper in a small bowl.

Assemble the Salad:

Arrange mixed greens on a serving platter.

Top with cooked potatoes, green beans, cherry tomatoes, Niçoise olives, capers, and tuna.

Drizzle the vinaigrette over the salad.

Season with salt and pepper to taste.

Serve the Tuna Niçoise salad immediately, garnished with the quartered hard-boiled eggs.

This Tuna Niçoise salad is a delicious and satisfying meal that combines protein-rich tuna with fresh vegetables and a tangy vinaigrette dressing. Enjoy!

Asian Quinoa Stir-Fry

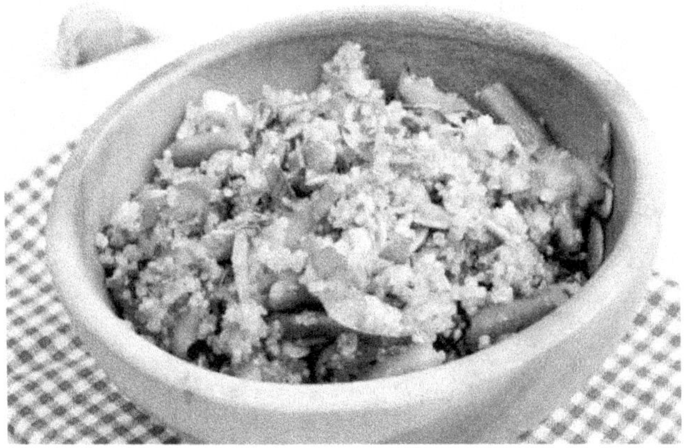

Ingredients:

2 cups Cooked quinoa

Mixed stir-fry vegetables (bell peppers, snap peas, carrots)

1 cup Tofu or chicken diced

1 tbsp Soy sauce

1 clove Garlic, minced

1 tsp Ginger, grated

Splash of Sesame oil

Instructions:

In a large pan, saute garlic and ginger in sesame oil.

Add the tofu or chicken and cook until browned.

Stir in the mixed vegetables and cook until tender.

Add cooked quinoa and soy sauce, and stir-fry until well combined.

Serve this flavorful Asian quinoa stir-fry for a filling and nutritious lunch.

Menopause-Friendly Vegetable Soup:

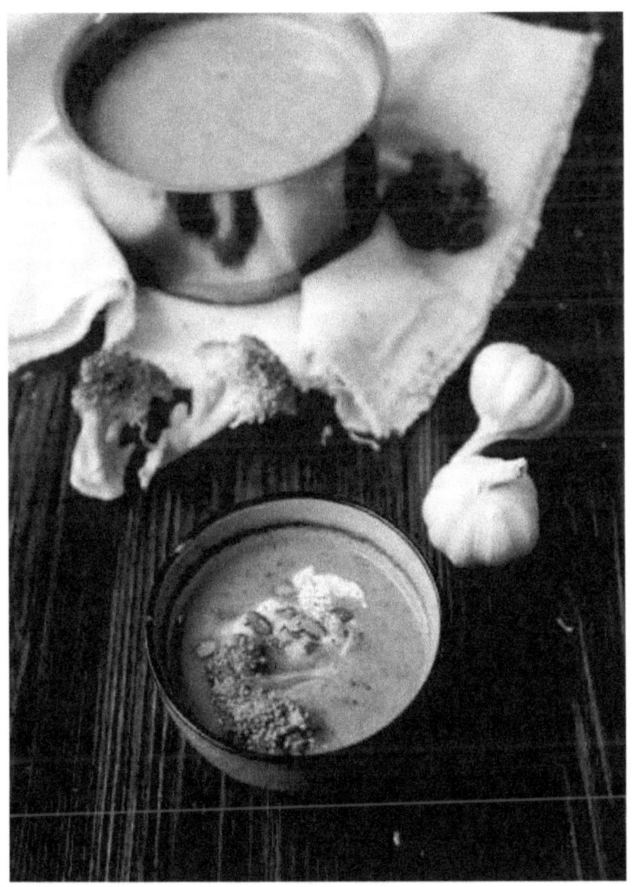

Ingredients:

1 tbsp olive oil

1 onion, diced

2 cloves garlic, minced

2 carrots, sliced

2 celery stalks, chopped

1 zucchini, diced

1 cup broccoli florets

6 cups vegetable broth

1 tsp turmeric powder

1 tsp ginger powder

1 tsp dried thyme

Salt and pepper to taste

Fresh parsley for garnish

Instructions:

Saute Aromatics:
Heat olive oil over medium heat in a large pot. Add diced onion and minced garlic.
Saute until fragrant.

Add Vegetables:
Add carrots, celery, zucchini, and broccoli to the pot.
Cook for a few minutes until slightly softened.

Season the Soup:
Pour in the vegetable broth and bring the soup to a simmer.
Stir in turmeric, ginger, and thyme. Season with salt and pepper to taste.

Simmer and Serve:

Let the soup simmer for 20-25 minutes until the vegetables are tender. Taste and adjust seasoning if needed. Serve the vegetable soup hot, garnished with fresh parsley. This vegetable soup contains nutrients and anti-inflammatory ingredients like turmeric and ginger that may help alleviate some menopause symptoms. It's a comforting and healthy option for a menopause-friendly meal. Feel free to customize the recipe by adding other vegetables or herbs based on your preferences. Enjoy!

Mediterranean Chickpea Salad

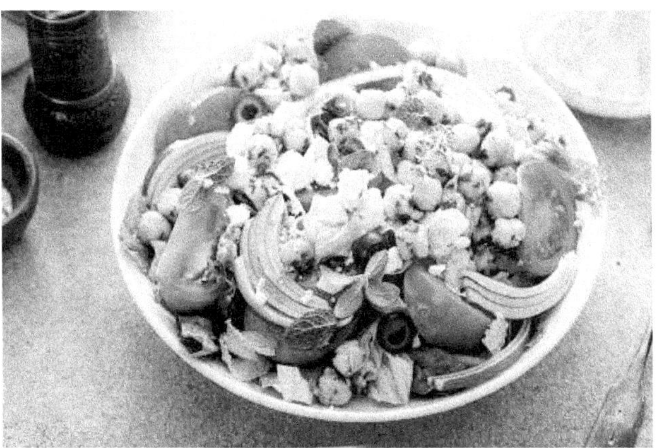

Ingredients:

1 Can of chickpeas, rinsed and drained

1/2 cup Cucumber, diced

1/2 cup Cherry tomatoes, halved

1/4 cup Kalamata olives, pitted

1/4 cup Red onion, thinly sliced

1/4 cup Feta cheese, crumbled

Lemon-herb vinaigrette

Fresh parsley, chopped

Salt and pepper

Instructions:

Combine chickpeas, cucumber, tomatoes, olives, red onion, and feta cheese in a bowl.

Drizzle with lemon-herb vinaigrette and toss gently to mix.

Garnish with chopped parsley and season with salt and pepper.

Serve this Mediterranean chickpea salad for a flavorful and protein-rich lunch.

Shrimp and Avocado taco

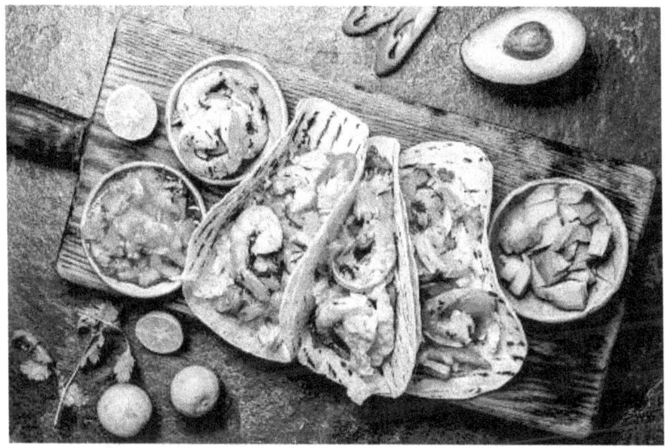

Ingredients:

Cooked shrimp, peeled and deveined

1 Avocado, sliced

1/2 cup Red cabbage, thinly sliced

1/4 cup Lime mayo (mayonnaise mixed with lime juice)

4 Whole grain wrap or tortilla

Fresh cilantro leaves

Salt and pepper

Instructions:

Spread lime mayo on the wrap.

Layer cooked shrimp, avocado slices, red cabbage, and cilantro leaves.

Season with salt and pepper, roll up the ingredients in the wrap and enjoy this light and zesty shrimp and avocado wrap.

Easy Burrito Bowl:

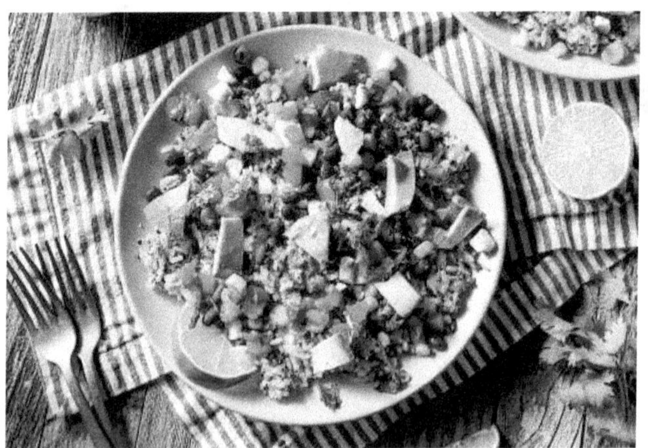

Ingredients:

1 cup cooked quinoa or rice

1 can black beans, drained and rinsed

1 cup corn kernels (canned or frozen)

1 avocado, sliced

1/2 cup cherry tomatoes, halved

1/2 cup diced bell peppers

1/4 cup diced red onion

Fresh cilantro for garnish

Lime wedges for serving

Instructions:

Prepare the Base:

Divide the cooked quinoa or rice into bowls.

Assemble the Bowl:

Add black beans, corn, avocado, cherry tomatoes, bell peppers, and red onion to the quinoa or rice.

Garnish and Serve:

Top with fresh cilantro.

Serve with lime wedges on the side for extra flavor.

Enjoy:

Mix all the ingredients in the bowl before eating for a delicious combination of flavors.

Squeeze lime juice over the bowl before enjoying it.

This Easy Burrito Bowl is a simple and nutritious meal.

Enjoy these lunch recipes for various flavors and nutrients in your midday meal!

Dinner Recipes: Learn how to prepare wholesome and satisfying dinner meals that promote relaxation and support restful sleep.

Easy Menopause-Friendly Thai Coconut Curry

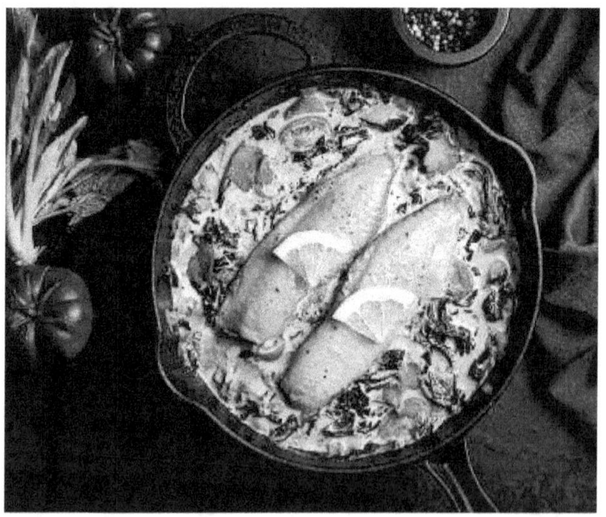

Ingredients:

4 salmon fillets

1 can (14 oz) light coconut milk

2 tbsps red curry paste

1 tbsp low-sodium soy sauce

1 tbsp honey or maple syrup

1 red bell pepper, sliced

1 small onion, sliced

1 tbsp coconut oil

Fresh cilantro for garnish Lime wedges for serving

Instructions:

Prepare the Curry Sauce:
In a large skillet, melt coconut oil over medium heat.
Add red curry paste and cook for a minute.
Pour in light coconut milk, soy sauce, and sweetener.
Stir well.

Cook the Salmon and Vegetables:
Place the salmon fillets in the curry sauce.
Cook for 5-6 minutes, flipping midway until the salmon is cooked.
Add sliced red bell pepper and onion to the skillet.
Cook for an additional 3-4 minutes until vegetables are tender.

This easy and flavorful Thai Coconut Curry Salmon recipe is a simple way to enjoy a delicious and nutritious meal that is beneficial during menopause.

Quinoa Stuffed Bell Peppers.

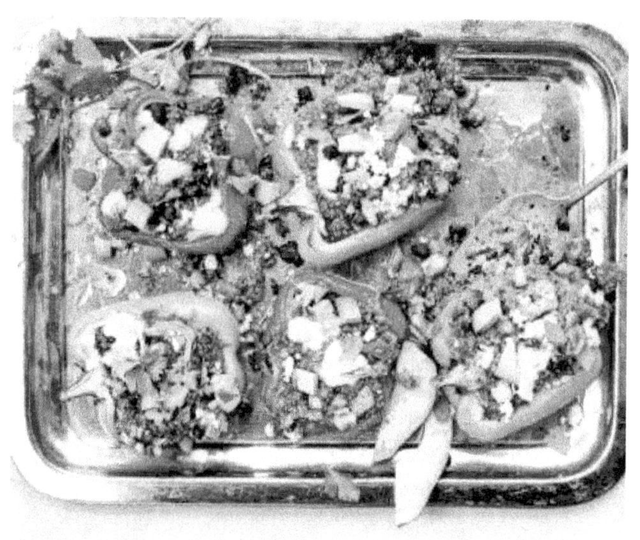

Ingredients:

4 bell peppers

1 cup cooked quinoa

1 can black beans, drained and rinsed

1 cup corn kernels

1/2 cup salsa

1/2 Avocado

1 tsp cumin

Salt and pepper to taste

Shredded cheese (optional)

Instructions:

Preheat the oven to 375°F (190°C) and prepare the bell peppers by cutting off the tops and removing the seeds.

Combine cooked quinoa, black beans, corn, salsa, cumin, salt, and pepper in a mixing bowl.

Stuff the bell peppers with the quinoa mixture.

Place the stuffed peppers in a baking dish, cover with foil, and bake for 25-30 minutes. Sprinkle with shredded cheese if desired before serving.

Balsamic Glazed Chicken with Roasted Vegetables

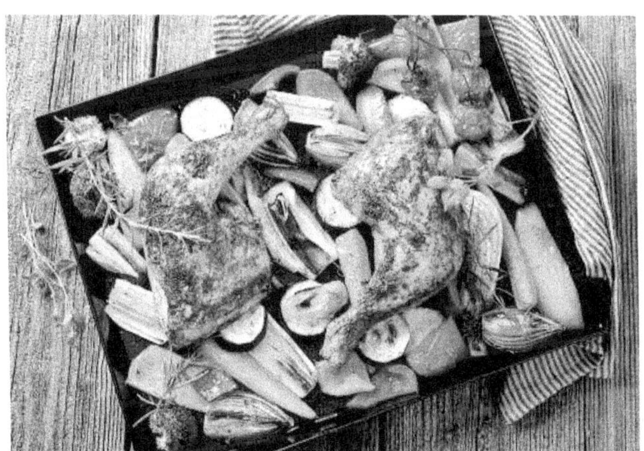

Ingredients:

2 boneless, skinless chicken breasts or legs

1/4 cup balsamic vinegar

2 tbsp honey

2 cloves garlic, minced

1 tsp dried rosemary

1 red onion

Mixed vegetables (bell peppers, zucchini, cherry tomatoes, carrot)

Olive oil

Salt and pepper to taste

Instructions:

Preheat the oven to 400°F (200°C) and line a baking sheet with parchment paper.

Mix balsamic vinegar, honey, garlic, and rosemary in a bowl.

Place the chicken breasts on the baking sheet and brush with the balsamic mixture.

Toss the mixed vegetables with olive oil, salt, and pepper, and spread them around the chicken.

Bake for 20-25 minutes or until chicken is cooked and vegetables are tender.

Lentil Bolognese with Zucchini Noodles

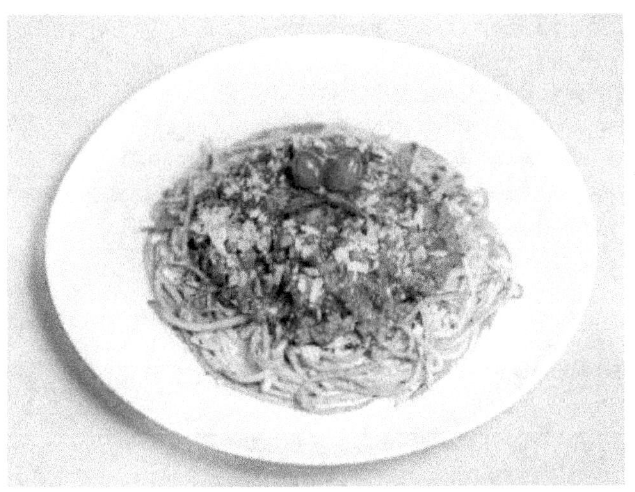

Ingredients:

1 cup cooked lentils

1 can crushed tomatoes

1 onion, diced

2 cloves garlic, minced

Italian seasoning

Zucchini spiraled into noodles

Olive oil

Salt and pepper to taste

Fresh basil, chopped (for garnish)

Instructions:

In a pan, sauté onion and garlic in olive oil until translucent.

Add cooked lentils and crushed tomatoes to the pan.

Season with Italian seasoning, salt, and pepper, and simmer for 15-20 minutes.

In another pan, cook zucchini noodles until slightly softened.

Serve the lentil Bolognese over zucchini noodles and garnish with fresh basil.

Tofu Stir-Fry with Brown Rice

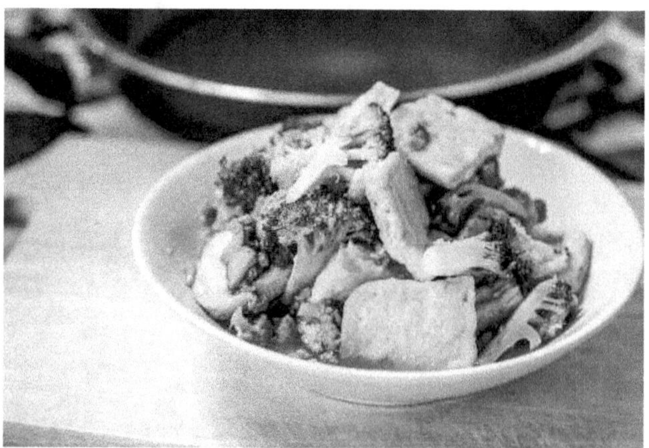

Ingredients:

1 block of firm tofu, cubed

Assorted stir-fry vegetables (such as bell peppers, broccoli, carrots)

Splash of Soy sauce

1/4 cup Ginger, minced

1 clove Garlic, minced

1 cup Brown rice, cooked

1 tbsp Sesame oil

Green onions, chopped (for garnish)

Instructions:

In a wok or large skillet, stir-fry tofu until golden brown.

Add vegetables, ginger, and garlic, and cook until vegetables are tender-crisp.

Drizzle with soy sauce and sesame oil.

Serve over brown rice and garnish with chopped green onions.

Easy Chicken Curry:

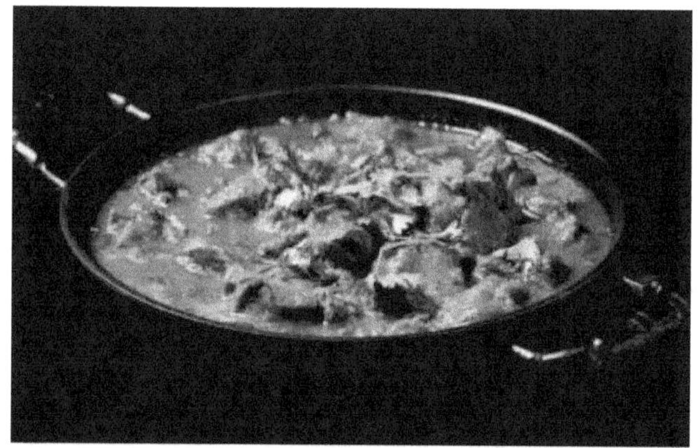

Ingredients:

4 chicken breast, cubed

1 tbsp vegetable oil

1 onion, chopped

2 cloves garlic, minced

2 tbsp curry powder

1 can diced tomatoes

1 can of coconut milk

Salt and pepper to taste

Instructions:

In a large pan, heat vegetable oil.

Add chicken and cook until browned.

Add onion, garlic, and curry powder.

Cook for a few minutes.

Pour in diced tomatoes and coconut milk.

Season with salt and pepper.

Simmer for about 45-60 minutes until beef is tender.

Serve hot and enjoy with whole-grain rice

This easy Chicken Curry is quick to make and full of delicious flavors. It's a perfect dish for a comforting and satisfying meal!

Lemon Garlic Shrimp and Asparagus

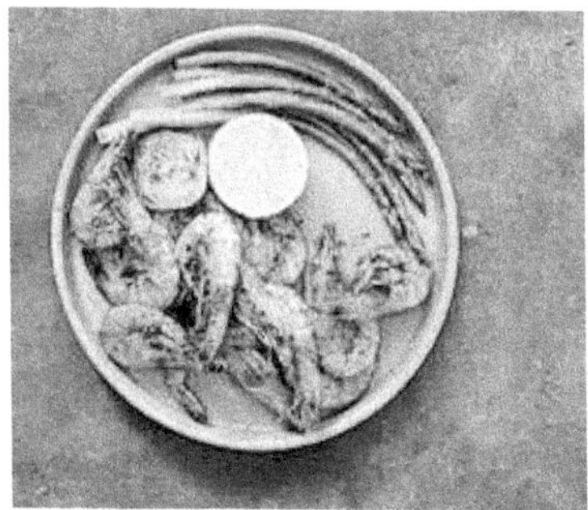

Ingredients:

1 lb shrimp, peeled and deveined

A bunch of asparagus, trimmed

Lemon juice and zest

2 cloves Garlic, minced

2 tbsps Olive oil

Salt and pepper

Instructions:

Preheat the oven to 400°F (200°C).

In a bowl, toss shrimp and asparagus with lemon zest, garlic, olive oil, salt, and pepper.

Spread on a baking sheet and roast for 12-15 minutes.

Squeeze lemon juice over the cooked shrimp and asparagus before serving.

Eggplant Parmesan

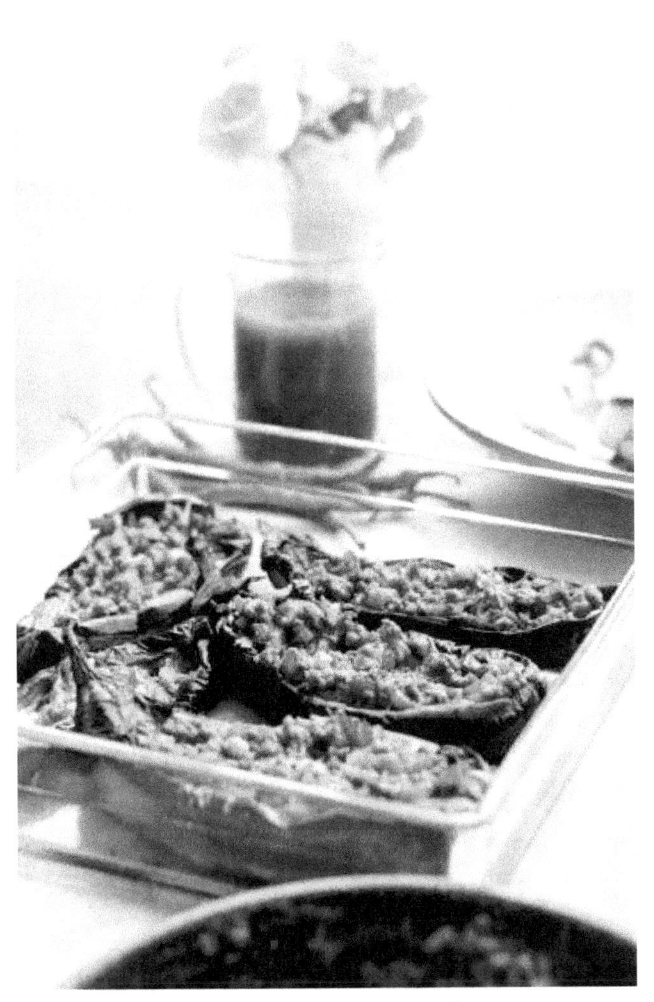

Ingredients:

2 large eggplant, sliced

2 tbsp Marinara sauce

1 cup Mozzarella cheese

1/2 cup Parmesan cheese

1/4 cup Italian breadcrumbs

Fresh basil

Olive oil

Salt and pepper

Instructions:

Preheat the oven to 375°F (190°C).

Dip eggplant slices in beaten egg and coat with breadcrumbs.

Bake until golden brown.

Layer eggplant slices with marinara sauce, cheese, and basil.

Repeat layers and bake until cheese is melted and bubbly.

Baked Salmon

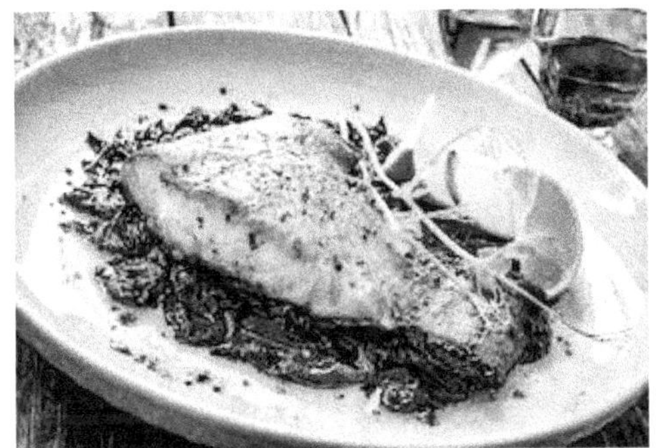

Ingredients:

4 salmon fillets

2 cups spinach

Lemon slices

1 tbsp Olive oil

1 clove Garlic, minced

Salt and pepper

Instructions:

Preheat the oven to 375°F (190°C) and line a baking dish with parchment paper.

Place salmon fillets in the dish on the spinach and lemon slices.

Mix olive oil, minced garlic, salt, and pepper in a small bowl.

Drizzle the olive oil mixture over the salmon and spinach.

Bake for 12-15 minutes or until the salmon is cooked through.

Garnish with fresh herbs before serving.

These recipes offer a variety of flavors and nutrients to support menopausal health through nutritious and delicious dinner options.

Stuffed Sweet Potatoes

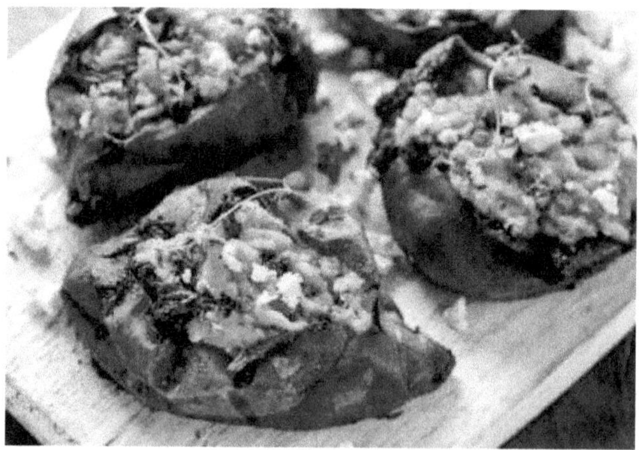

Ingredients:

4 medium sweet potatoes

Avocado, diced

Red onion, diced

crumble of feta cheese

Fresh cilantro, chopped

Lime juice

Cumin, paprika, salt, and pepper

Instructions:

Preheat the oven to 400°F (200°C) and prick sweet potatoes with a fork.

Bake sweet potatoes for 45-60 minutes until tender.

Mix the red onion, cilantro, lime juice, and spices in a bowl.

Split sweet potatoes open and stuff them with the mixture. Garnish with additional cilantro and feta, and serve with a side salad.

Snack Suggestions: Explore healthy snack ideas to curb cravings and provide additional nutrients between meals for optimal menopausal health.

Here are some healthy snack suggestions tailored for menopause to keep you energized and satisfied in between meals:

- **Greek Yogurt with Berries:** Serve Greek yogurt topped with fresh berries, such as blueberries, strawberries, or raspberries. Greek yogurt is rich in protein and probiotics, while berries provide antioxidants and vitamins.
- **Nut Butter Apple Slices:** Slice up an apple and spread almond or peanut butter on each slice. Apples offer fiber and natural sweetness, while nut butter adds healthy fats and protein to keep you full.
- **Mixed Nuts and Dried Fruit:** Create your trail mix by combining unsalted mixed nuts like almonds, walnuts, and cashews with dried fruit such as apricots, raisins, or cranberries. This snack balances protein, healthy fats, and natural sugars.
- **Vegetable Hummus Dip:** Dip baby carrots, cucumber slices, bell pepper strips, or cherry tomatoes in hummus for a crunchy and satisfying snack. Hummus is a good source of plant-based protein, while vegetables offer fiber and essential nutrients.
- **Rice Cake with Avocado:** Top a rice cake with mashed avocado, a sprinkle of sea salt, and a drizzle of olive oil. Avocado provides healthy fats and fiber, while rice cakes offer a light and crunchy base.
- **Hard-Boiled Egg with Whole-Grain Crackers:** Enjoy a hard-boiled egg with a few whole-grain crackers for a protein-rich, portable snack. Eggs are a source of high-quality protein; whole-grain crackers add fiber and complex carbohydrates.
- **Cottage Cheese with Pineapple:** For a balanced snack, serve cottage cheese topped with pineapple chunks. Cottage cheese offers protein and calcium, while pineapple adds a sweet, tangy flavor and vitamin C.
- **Chia Pudding:** Make chia pudding by mixing chia seeds with almond milk and a touch of honey or maple syrup. Let it sit in the fridge until it thickens, then top with sliced fruits or nuts for a nutritious and filling snack. These snack suggestions provide a mix of nutrients to fuel your body and help you manage hunger and energy levels between meals during menopause.
- **Edamame Beans:** Enjoy a serving of steamed edamame beans sprinkled with sea salt. These soybeans are a good source of plant-based protein, fiber, and essential nutrients, making them a satisfying and nutritious snack.
- **Celery Sticks with Almond Butter:** Spread almond butter on celery sticks for a crunchy and easy snack. Celery is low in calories and water content, while almond butter provides healthy fats and protein, creating a satisfying combination.
- **Yogurt Parfait with Granola:** Layer Greek yogurt with granola and mixed berries in a glass for a wholesome and tasty snack. Greek yogurt offers protein and probiotics, granola provides fiber and crunch, and berries add antioxidants and natural sweetness.

- **Quinoa Salad Cups:** Fill mini lettuce cups with a quinoa salad made with cooked quinoa, diced veggies, chickpeas, and a lemon-tahini dressing. These bite-sized quinoa cups are a balanced and flavorful snack option.
- **Cucumber Tuna Boats**: Hollow out cucumber halves and fill them with tuna salad made with canned tuna, Greek yogurt, diced celery, and lemon juice. These refreshing cucumber boats offer protein, hydration, and crunch in one convenient snack.
- **Dark Chocolate-Covered Almonds:** Indulge in a small portion of dark chocolate-covered almonds for a sweet and satisfying treat. Dark chocolate provides antioxidants, while almonds offer healthy fats and a crunch, creating a delightful snack with a hint of sweetness.
- **Berry Smoothie:** Blend mixed berries, Greek yogurt, almond milk, and a handful of spinach for a refreshing and nutrient-packed smoothie. This smoothie provides fiber, vitamins, and antioxidants and is a delicious snack.
- **Roasted Chickpeas:** Roast chickpeas with olive oil and seasoning until crispy for a crunchy and protein-rich snack. These roasted chickpeas offer fiber and plant-based protein, making them a satisfying and healthy dietary choice.

These snack suggestions provide a mix of nutrients to fuel your body and help you manage hunger and energy levels between meals during menopause.

Embarking on the **seven-day menopause diet** and implementing strategies for hormonal balance sets a strong foundation for resetting your hormones and setting you up for long-term well-being. You are taking proactive steps toward achieving and maintaining hormonal harmony by nourishing your body with nutrient-dense foods, adopting healthy lifestyle practices, and prioritizing self-care. This initial commitment to resetting your hormones is a powerful start to cultivating a balanced and thriving internal environment, supporting overall health and vitality during the menopausal transition.

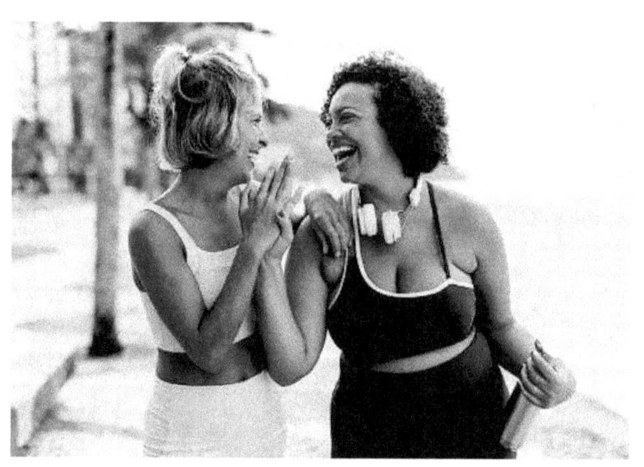

Menopause Mind:

- **Mindfulness Practices:** Incorporate mindfulness meditation, deep breathing exercises, or journalism into your daily routine to promote mental clarity and emotional well-being.
- **Emotional Support:** Seek professional help from therapists or counselors to address and navigate the emotional changes that may accompany menopause, fostering a supportive environment for mental health.

Body:

- **Physical Activity:** To promote physical strength and flexibility during menopause, choose activities that suit your fitness level, such as yoga, walking, or strength training.
- **Sleep Hygiene:** Establish a bedtime routine that encourages restful sleep, creating an environment conducive to hormonal balance and overall health.
- **Nutrient-Dense Diet:** Nourish your body with whole foods rich in nutrients essential for hormonal health, hydration, and vitality.
- **Soul:Self-Compassion:** Practice self-care and self-compassion by setting boundaries, prioritizing activities that bring joy, and honoring your emotional needs.

During the menopausal transition, caring for your **mind, body,** and **soul** becomes paramount in maintaining overall well-being. To nurture your mind, consider incorporating stress-reducing practices such as mindfulness meditation, deep breathing exercises, or journalism to cultivate mental clarity and emotional resilience. Engaging in activities that bring joy and fulfillment, such as hobbies, spending time with loved ones, or pursuing creative outlets, can also contribute to positive mental health during this transformative phase. Additionally, seeking professional support from therapists or counselors can provide a safe space to address any emotional challenges or changes that may arise during menopause. For your body, prioritize physical activity that suits your fitness level and preferences, whether through gentle yoga, brisk walks, strength training, or any exercise that promotes strength and flexibility. Adequate sleep is crucial for hormonal balance, so establish a bedtime routine that encourages restful sleep and consider creating a comfortable sleep environment. Nourish your body with whole, nutrient-dense foods that support hormonal health, hydration, and overall well-being. Lastly, for your soul, practice self-compassion and self-care by setting boundaries, saying no when needed, and prioritizing activities that nurture your spirit, such as mindfulness practices, spending time in nature, or engaging in spiritual practices that resonate with you. Embracing a holistic approach to caring for your **mind, body,** and **soul** can empower you to navigate the menopausal journey with grace and resilience.

Staying hydrated is crucial during menopause, as adequate water intake supports hormonal balance, regulates body temperature, and helps alleviate symptoms like hot flashes and dry skin. Moreover, water plays a significant role in weight loss by promoting satiety, boosting metabolism, and aiding in the digestion and absorption of nutrients. Opting for water-rich fruits can be a refreshing and flavorful way to increase your fluid intake while reaping the benefits of essential vitamins, minerals, and antioxidants. Incorporating infused water with fruits adds natural flavor and provides a hydrating and nourishing option to support overall health and well-being during the menopausal transition.

List of Fruit-Infused Water Ideas:

- **Strawberry and Mint:** Sliced strawberries and fresh mint leaves add flavor to your water, enhancing its taste and providing antioxidants.
- **Cucumber and Lemon:** Cucumber slices paired with lemon wedges create a refreshing and detoxifying drink that can help flush out toxins and support hydration.
- **Orange and Blueberry:** Oranges and blueberries infused in water offer a citrus and sweet blend rich in vitamin C and antioxidants, promoting skin health and immune support.
- **Watermelon and Basil:** Watermelon chunks with basil leaves result in a hydrating and revitalizing drink that is both refreshing and hydrating.
- **Lime and Raspberry:** Fresh lime juice mixed with raspberries creates a zesty concoction that adds flavor to your water while providing vitamin C and fiber.

List of Vitamins and Supplements for Menopause:

- **Vitamin D :** Supports bone health and immune function, especially during menopause, when bone density may decrease.
- **Calcium:** Is essential for maintaining bone strength and density and helping to prevent osteoporosis, a common concern during and after menopause.
- **Vitamin B Complex:** Supports energy production, mood regulation, and cognitive function, which can be beneficial for managing menopausal symptoms.
- **Omega-3 Fatty Acids:** Promote heart health, reduce inflammation, and support brain function, potentially easing menopausal symptoms like mood swings.
- **Magnesium:** Aids in muscle relaxation, stress reduction, and quality sleep, which can be beneficial for managing menopausal symptoms such as insomnia and anxiety.
- **Black Cohosh:** Herbal supplement used to alleviate hot flashes, night sweats, and mood fluctuations commonly experienced during menopause
- **Evening Primrose Oil:** Contains gamma-linolenic acid (GLA) that may help reduce menopausal symptoms like breast tenderness and mood swings.

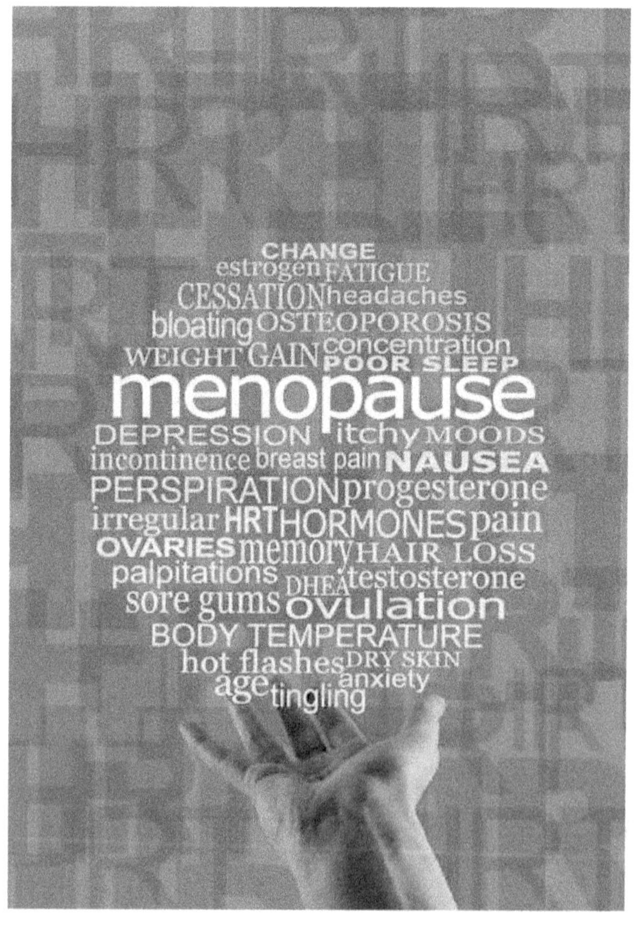

CHANGE
estrogen FATIGUE
CESSATION headaches
bloating OSTEOPOROSIS
concentration
WEIGHT GAIN POOR SLEEP
menopause
DEPRESSION itchy MOODS
incontinence breast pain NAUSEA
PERSPIRATION progesterone
irregular HRT HORMONES pain
OVARIES memory HAIR LOSS
palpitations DHEA testosterone
sore gums ovulation
BODY TEMPERATURE
hot flashes DRY SKIN
age tingling anxiety

Conclusion

In conclusion, the "7-Day Menopause Diet" offers more than just a meal plan – it provides a blueprint for embracing menopause with vitality and wellness. Throughout this journey, the focus has been on nourishing the body, supporting hormonal balance, and fostering a sense of empowerment through mindful eating. Following this structured plan, women can embark on a path toward improved health, increased energy, and a renewed sense of well-being during menopause. Each day of the "7-Day Menopause Diet" has been carefully crafted to offer nutritious and delicious meals that cater to the unique needs of menopausal women. From nutrient-dense breakfasts to satisfying lunches and flavorful dinners, this book has aimed to elevate the dining experience while addressing menopausal symptoms and supporting overall health. As you reach the end of this transformative week, I encourage you to reflect on the impact of these dietary changes on your body and mind. Embrace the knowledge from this meal plan as a tool for long-term well-being and vitality. Remember that every choice you make in nourishing your body is a step towards a healthier and happier menopausal experience. Your feedback is invaluable. If the "7-Day Menopause Diet" has resonated with you and made a positive difference in your menopausal journey, please consider leaving a review on Amazon. Your review can guide and inspire other women seeking to navigate menopause with grace, balance, and health-conscious choices. Thank you for embarking on this week-long menopausal nutritional experience. May the principles and recipes shared in the "7-Day Menopause Diet" continue to nourish and support you on your path to wellness and vitality during this transformative phase of life. Here's to embracing menopause with strength, resilience, and a newfound appreciation for the power of food.

Reference

If you're looking for reliable information on menopause, I recommend checking reputable sources such as:

Mayo Clinic - Menopause:Website: https://www.mayoclinic.org/diseases-conditions/menopause/symp toms-causes/syc-20353397

National Institute on Aging - Menopause:Website: https://www.nia.nih.gov/health/menopause .

American College of Obstetricians and Gynecologists - Menopause FAQs:Website: https://www.acog.org/womens-health/faqs/menopause .

For support, advice, and information on nutrition and well-being during menopause, you can contact healthcare professionals, nutritionists, mental health counselors, and women's health organizations. Additionally, online communities and forums focused on menopause can provide valuable insights and support from individuals going through similar experiences. Remember that you must consult with healthcare providers or specialists for personalized recommendations and guidance tailored to your specific health needs and concerns during the menopause transition.